I0116867

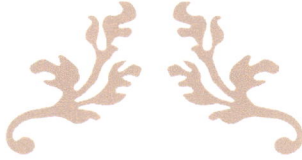

CANCER WAS OUR BLESSING

By Yolanda Commack

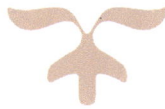

Introduction

Yolanda Commack, AKA Lonnie Bush, is the author of, *Cancer Was My Blessing*. In her book, Lonnie shares her testimony of battling triple negative Breast Cancer, and all the ups and downs that came along with her diagnosis. The more speaking engagements she accepted as a Breast Cancer spokesperson, the more she realized that the stories of other survivors needed to be shared. She became an advocate for the women she encountered and began asking the women she met to keep journals of their good days, tough days, and everyday life after their diagnosis. Lonnie also asked the family members of the women who had lost the battle to share stories on behalf of their loved ones. Cancer is scary, frustrating, and confusing. It makes some going through the battle stronger, and also destroys some relationships. In some instances, it even creates new friendships, and life-long bonds. As with any war, some win the fight, and others lose. No matter what God allows, we must accept and pray for peace and understanding!

Going through her own personal experience with Cancer was only half the battle for Lonnie. Instead of wallowing in what was happening to her, she kept the faith and encouraged others along the way. Through it all, Lonnie learned to accept that Cancer wasn't a curse, it was her blessing!

Achieving My Dreams After Diagnosis

If you keep the faith, and trust God and His word, His promises will come to pass. Yes, things are going to be rough at times; He didn't promise you that life would be easy. He promised that He would never leave or forsake you. I reminded myself of that, even in the hard times.

One of my goals in life was to have my own gym. Even with my diagnosis, I wasn't going to give up that dream. I had my eye on a location and came close to buying it. A friend, who is mentioned in my last book, *Cancer Was My Blessing*, was supposed to help me secure a grant for the gym, but he never did. I was a little discouraged, but continued to stay faithful and believed that God would handle my situation. I gathered my thoughts, realizing that blessings delayed are not blessings denied. I knew I would have my gym one day, I just had to be patient and wait on God.

On May 31, 2013, I opened the doors to my very own fitness center in a better location than the one I was trying to obtain. God delivered, just like He said he would, and with over a hundred clients and four instructors; all while I was laid off from my job. I say that not to brag, but to say, "Look at God!"

"Don't take your eyes off Him and watch what happens."

As I continue on this blessed journey of mine, my Goal is to somehow secure a grant that will tie my love for fitness and my love for assisting Cancer patients together. I would love to have a gym big enough to have everything Cancer patients need such as wigs, hats, scarves, a steam room, and to be able to give them vouchers to pay for medication and copays; which many women can't afford. I also want to start support groups for the husbands and children of these women because they have no one to talk to about what they deal with while their wife or mother is battling Cancer. I'd also like to be able to assist financially for maid services or someone to run errands for Cancer patients, since they often don't have the time, energy or resources for minor things like that.

My love for fitness and a need to help my clients have the healthiest life possible, leads me to want a bigger gym than the one I have, so that I can incorporate more forms of working out, ropes, bikes, equipment and things like that. At some point, when I get a bigger gym, I want to offer classes specifically designed for Cancer patients. In the Raytown area, there aren't any gyms doing what I'm doing. I want to offer health and fitness counseling, which can address the issues of dealing with weight gain, because many of my clients are depressed, worried, or stressed, and it causes them to overeat. I would also love to purchase a van to pick up patients who need a ride to doctor appointments or grocery shopping.

My dreams are big. My desire to help others fight the ultimate fight is even bigger. I want to do so much, and when God gets ready to bless me, it will happen with the right grant and the help of the right person.

"I'm staying excited about life through all my ups and downs."

Acknowledgments

First, I'd like to thank God for all His blessings and grace. I could do nothing without Him! Second, I'd like to thank my parents for always believing in me, accepting me and loving me unconditionally. To my beautiful children: Koreyon and Trinity, thanks for sharing me with the world. Please know that everything I do is for you! My beautiful favorite sister, Tonia, who supports everything I do – I love you! To my brothers and sisters, thanks for loving me and my children.

To my LBF Crew, I could do absolutely nothing without you guys. God couldn't have blessed me with a better support team. Thanks for all the hours of loading and unloading, cleaning, planning, running, and all the things necessary to help me on a daily basis!

Kana (Soft Hands), Melvin (Fat Boy), Kita (Gayle), Nika (Booty Shake), and my nephew Keith, thanks for everything you do to support me. It baffles me, and I thank you from the bottom of my Heart!

Trisha Rushing, thanks for believing in my dreams! To all the hospitals and nurses that allowed me to come in and work with Cancer patients, and to all my clients that trust me...thank you!

To all my co-workers at Ford (too many to name), thanks for the support and love! Special thanks to all the book clubs and churches that promoted my first book, *Cancer Was My Blessing*.

A heartfelt thanks to my adopted mom Joyce, who accepted me as her daughter after I lost my beloved mom Christine Bush! To my cousin Kim (Cry Baby), thanks for always loving and checking on me! Thanks to my church home, Beacon Hills Church of the Nazarene. And a special, special, thanks to all my social media friends (*Twitter, Facebook, Instagram*), for following me and purchasing my books and DVDs. Last, but not least, I humbly thank anyone that I missed. Please charge it to my small memory and not my Big Heart!!

I love each and every one of you!

Thanks to all the individuals that shared their stories, and a special thanks to the families that shared stories from the women who have lost the *Battle,* but not the *Fight*!

~ Lonnie ~

Warrior Stories

Cancer Was OUR Blessing

We don't get to choose the path for our lives. It is chosen for us. No one would willingly choose a diagnosis of having Cancer, and those afflicted with the disease often ask, "Why me?" I know I asked myself that very question, and the answer never came. But I realized that sometimes the things in life that we have to go through, are put upon us so that we can make a difference in someone else's life. Sometimes the strength that we possess when dealing with hardships is just what someone else needs to witness in order to be stronger in dealing with hardships of their own.

Life is hard sometimes, and when it is, the only thing that we can control is our reaction to the hand that we are dealt. My blessings have been bountiful, and among them has been the opportunity to meet some of the strongest women I know. Adversity may have joined them on life's journey, but each and every one of them did not let Cancer change who they were. Getting to know them inspired me, and their stories are worthy to be shared.

Cancer Was OUR Blessing

Dana's Denial

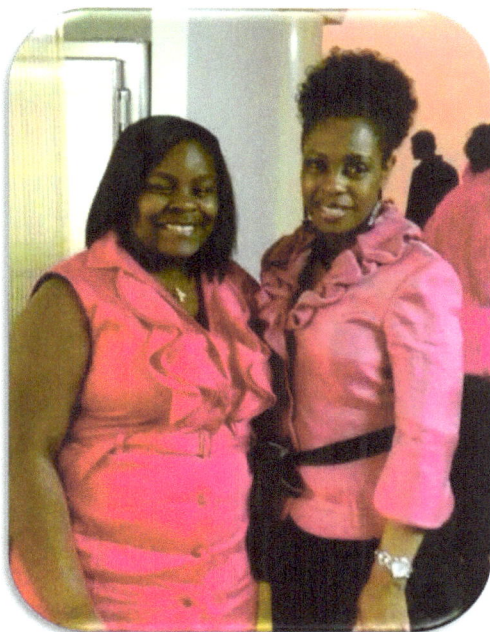

I met Lonnie Bush in November of 2010. I was referred to her by my husband. He and my daughter had been working out with Lonnie for about a year. I decided that I would try her fitness class since my normal class had cancelled several sessions. I took my friend Keisha with me. I remember it like it was yesterday. Lonnie was preparing the class to do a full body workout with eight-pound weights. Everyone knows that if you are a "New friend" of Lonnie's, she will cut you some slack on your first day. That was not so in my case! She looked at my friend Keisha and said, "Hi friend," and gave her some five-pound weights to use for her first Lonnie experience. She then looked at me and said, "You look strong," and put a pair of eight-pound weights in my hands! *Oh my God!*

Cancer Was OUR Blessing

The class definitely was not easy, and the pace was extremely fast. I loved it! On January 1, 2011, I became a permanent client of Lonnie Bush. Yes, you read that right, she does offer classes on New Year's Day.

You know how you always hear people say that God puts people in your life for a reason, well I truly believe that God did that for me when He allowed me to meet Lonnie. When Lonnie Bush becomes your trainer, you don't just work out. You do several fundraisers and charitable walks for Breast Cancer a year. We also participated in several Breast Cancer awareness events. Why does she do so many things for Breast Cancer? Because, she is a Breast Cancer survivor and is passionate about using her personal experience as a testimony for women who may be battling or about to start battling.

Well, while attending Lonnie's Breast Cancer awareness events and learning some of the signs of Breast Cancer, I had a strange experience of my own. I woke up one morning with blood on my sheets and my night shirt. It looked like it was coming from my right breast. I looked at my right breast closely, and it looked like it was coming from my nipple. I noticed that the skin around the areola was dry and crusty. Since, I struggle with eczema, I thought that the skin condition had just chosen to flare up on my nipple, so I moisturized it and went on about my day. Well, it kept happening. I would not only see the blood on my sheets, but on my bra as well. Still thinking that eczema was the culprit, I called my dermatologist and scheduled an appointment. My dermatologist looked at it and said that it looked like it could be eczema, but if the medicine he prescribed me did not work, then it may be something hormonal.

I had the prescription filled and began using it. The dryness, flakiness and itchiness went away completely after about a week, however, I was still waking up with blood on my sheets and night clothes. When I took my bra off at the end of the day, there was always still blood on it. I began to get nervous and very concerned. My breast tissue was naturally lumpy, and I had not been doing my monthly breast checks on a regular basis to get familiar with how they felt when they were normal, therefore, I was not able to feel any lumps, but when I squeezed my right nipple, blood was still coming out.

I had already scheduled an appointment with my gynecologist's office for my annual well-woman's checkup. I was not scheduled to see my regular gynecologist. Instead, I was scheduled to see a nurse practitioner. I explained to her what had been going on with my right breast for the last ninety days. She gave me a thorough manual breast exam, and stated that she felt a lump. She immediately sent me to get some blood work done, and before I left the office, I had an appointment with a breast surgeon. I met with the breast surgeon that same week. I had three mammograms and an ultrasound done. A procedure was also done where a needle was stuck into my nipple. It released a dye into my breast to help the doctor find out what was causing the bleeding. The procedure was very uncomfortable. After all of the tests were completed, it was determined that I had three lumps in my right breast, and a wart was causing all of the bleeding.

Surgery was scheduled to remove the wart. On the day of the surgery, I asked my doctor to look at the wart and tell me if it was Cancerous or not once they removed it. The procedure was an outpatient surgery, and before I was released, the doctor told me that the wart was not Cancerous. When I asked her about the three lumps that were found, she stated that my breast tissue would reabsorb those lumps in due time, so I went for my follow up appointments to make sure that I was healing properly from the surgery. The surgeon stated that everything looked good and released me from her care. I left the surgeon's office thinking that

I would never have to see her again. My problem had been solved, and no Cancer was found. *Right?*

Thanking God, I began to go about my everyday life. My daughter, Triniti, was on dance team and it was time to start preparing her for recital. I've been doing dance recitals with Triniti since she was three years old. I continued to work out with Lonnie, and I ran in the 5k race for my company in the annual KC Corporate Challenge. I had a personal best time of completing the race in thirty minutes. Yes, life was good and it was business as usual. I felt like God was really smiling down on me. He allowed me, and my ex-husband at the time, to mend our relationship and remarry in October of 2011. *Life was good!* But, there was just one thing, I still kept feeling the lump on the right side of my breast. Yes, the same breast that I had just had surgery on earlier that year. I would feel the lump and convince myself that it was nothing; after all, the doctor had told me that my breast tissue would reabsorb the lumps.

I would feel the lump on the side of my right breast every day. One day it felt bigger and began to hurt. I then began to talk about it with my husband. We started to think of other things that it could be. Maybe it was just fatty tissue, like a Lipoma. I reminded myself of one of Lonnie's Breast Cancer awareness events where a nurse was telling her story about a lump she had found in her breast and how she kept trying to explain it away.

I was led to go to Lonnie's place, one Friday evening after work to talk to her about it. If you ever talk to Lonnie about any type of lump, her first words will always be to have the doctor biopsy it, or just plain cut it out. I guess I just needed to hear somebody say it. I had already scheduled an appointment with my primary care physician in November of 2011. I went to the appointment. I explained to the doctor my concerns with my right breast. She gave me orders to get an ultrasound that same day. I got the ultrasound done, and the radiology technician told me that he could see the lump that I had been feeling. When I went back for my follow up appointment in December, I asked the doctor what I should do. She told me to follow up on it with my next mammogram. *My next mammogram! Wow!* I was not due for another mammogram until March. Well, I told myself, *she doesn't seem to be too worried about it so, I won't worry about it either.* Deep down inside I really didn't want to know, so it was easy to go on about my everyday life.

My life was business as usual. I went to work every day. I took Triniti back and forth to dance team practice and I helped her get ready for the upcoming dance competition in March. Preparing Triniti for competition was very time consuming, so I didn't take the time to schedule an appointment for a mammogram in March like I was supposed to. I had a business trip in May for work. I was trying to support my son by attending some of his track meets. After the March competition, I had to start getting Triniti ready for her dance recital in June. My life did not calm down enough for me to even think about scheduling an appointment for a mammogram until July. During all that time, I would wake up and feel the lump. I would take a shower and feel the lump. I would put clothes on and feel the lump. When I took off my clothes, I would feel the lump. I was worried about it, but I would push my worry to the side because I had way too much to do.

Triniti's dance recital was over, school was out, and things were finally starting to slow down. I finally remembered that I hadn't scheduled my mammogram, so I took time out to call and schedule the appointment. When I called to make the appointment, the scheduler asked me if I had any lumps. I told her yes, one on the side of my right breast that I could feel. She informed that me that I would also have to get an ultrasound done since I was able to feel a lump. The appointment was scheduled for the last week of July 2012. Yes, that's right July 2012, about eight months from the last time I saw my primary care provider, and four months from the time I should have scheduled my follow up mammogram for March.

The day came for my mammogram. Both the mammogram and the ultrasound were done. I was told to wait in the waiting room, and was given the option of a foot massage or a body massage on an automated massage table while I waited. I didn't even have a chance to choose which massage I wanted before the nurse came back in the room. When she came back in, she had a very serious look on her face, and asked me with a sense of urgency in her voice if I had a mammogram back in 2010. I advised her that I had and that it was performed at my job. We had a health fair in 2010 and there was a mobile mammogram machine from St. Luke's Hospital there, and that is where I had my mammogram done that year. They had filed for payment for the visit through my insurance company, and sent me a letter notifying me that my mammogram came back normal.

After all of the commotion in the doctor's office, and the worried look on the nurse's face, I really needed a massage. I was truly stressed! They didn't say that I had Cancer, but there was definitely a problem. I could tell it by their actions. They wanted to see the letter St. Luke's had sent to me. I advised them that the mammogram had been done two years ago, and I no longer had the letter that they sent me.

The doctor urged me to make an appointment with my breast surgeon right away. So, I did. I also received a letter from them in just a couple days, advising me that they had found something in my breast and that I needed to follow up with my doctor. Well, I immediately called my breast surgeon. I advised them of the results of my mammogram and scheduled an appointment for that same week.

Cancer Was OUR Blessing

I went in for a biopsy of the lump on my right breast. They used the ultrasound machine to find the lump, and the radiology technician marked it for the doctor to be able to see it more easily to perform the biopsy. They gave me some medicine to numb the pain, and she took several samples of the tissue from the lump. My surgeon said that she would have her nurse call me with the results. Before the doctor left the room I asked her, "I thought you said that my breast tissue would reabsorb all three of the lumps." She didn't have much to say about her previous statement. She did say, however, that she did not expect the lump that we had just biopsied to be Cancerous.

So I left the hospital and went on about my life; business as usual. The only person who knew about the biopsy was my husband. I pushed the possibility of having breast Cancer to the back of my mind. I still didn't really think that it could happen to me. I received the call on a Friday morning concerning the biopsy results. I was at work. The call was different than the normal follow-up calls in that the call was not from my surgeon's nurse, it was from my surgeon herself. She asked me if it was a good time to talk. I told her to hold on and to give me time to step away from my desk. My heart was literally in my throat. The doctor doesn't normally call if everything is okay. When things are fine, you get a call from a nurse, or a letter stating that everything is good. As I went to a place where I could have a little privacy, I knew that a personal call from the doctor could not be good news.

The doctor proceeds to tell me that the lump that I had been so carefully watching and ignoring for almost a year, was a Cancerous tumor. I would like to say that I was totally thrown off guard or blindsided, but I wasn't. Deep down inside I knew something was wrong the whole time. I just didn't want to believe it. Even hearing the doctor tell me I had Breast Cancer did not make it seem any more real to me. I scheduled another appointment with my surgeon to discuss the different options I had to choose from in order to get rid of the Cancer. After I hung up with my surgeon, I met with my immediate supervisor and the director of my department. I told them that I had been diagnosed with Stage 1 Breast Cancer and needed to take the rest of the day off to wrap my mind around the diagnosis and to be with my family. I also asked that they not share the diagnosis with the rest of my team. I didn't want anyone feeling sorry for me or treating me differently.

I called my husband and told him the results of the biopsy. He was shocked! He really did believe that what was going on in my breast was something minor. I then called my mom to let her know. I thank God every day for my mother. She immediately told me not to worry, and that she would be with me throughout the whole process. I waited for my husband to come home so that we could tell our children together. My daughter was twelve years old at the time, but she had attended several Breast Cancer awareness events and understood the seriousness of the diagnosis. My son had just turned eighteen years old and was about to be a senior in high school. I am not sure if he understood the seriousness of the diagnosis. Myles didn't really have any questions, but Triniti had a ton of questions. We ended the conversation with hugs, kisses, and telling each other that we love them.

My husband caused my day to end on a positive note. As he held me in his arms, he told me that everything was going to be alright. He did not believe that God had allowed us to remarry, only to take me away from him. He just knew that God would not leave him alone to raise our awesome, but sometimes challenging, daughter by himself. We both laughed ourselves to sleep about that idea.

The next day before work out class, I told Lonnie about the diagnosis. She was upset and said out loud how much she hated Cancer. She gave me a hug and asked everyone that was there to make a circle and hold hands while she prayed for me concerning the battle that I was about to go through. I received her prayer, but I had no idea of what laid ahead of me. Lonnie had some idea, but everyone's battle is different. I wasn't sure at that time if I wanted everyone to know about my diagnosis. I just didn't want people to treat me differently, but the shout outs on her Facebook page, and the hugs people gave me, really made me feel good to know that someone else besides my immediate family also cared.

The following weeks were filled with doctor's appointments and tests. Lonnie and my mom went with me to my first appointment with my surgeon to discuss the diagnosis and my options. Lonnie was able to help me ask better questions since she had already been through the process. The surgeon advised me of my options and advised me that the type of Cancer I had was a slow-growing Cancer, and that it was not aggressive. It was called Invasive Ductal

Carcinoma of the breast. This Cancer was hormonal, just like my dermatologist had suspected. The tumor was still considered to be Stage 1, and it was inside the duct of my right breast. The first test that I took was a comprehensive BRAC Analysis test. The test consisted of me swishing mouthwash around in my mouth and spitting into a cup. They would send the cup to the lab to determine the results. The BRAC test would tell the doctors whether the Cancer I had was hereditary or not. I was very concerned about the results of this test because I did not want my daughter to have to worry about being affected by Breast Cancer.

Before I left my first appointment, an MRI had been scheduled for that same week. They were doing the MRI to make sure that there was no Cancer in any other part of my body. The time came for me to go and get the MRI done. Unfortunately, my mother was not able to go with me. She was not able to give enough advance notice to her job to get off work for the appointment, so my mother-in-law and daughter volunteered to go with me. The radiology technician came to get me from the waiting room, and she asked if my daughter and mother-in-law wanted to come to the area where the test was going to be done, but they declined. I changed my clothes and put on the "all too familiar" to me by now, hospital gown. The lady that was doing the MRI started explaining to me what the test would consist of. She told me that I would have to lay very still on a narrow table inside the MRI machine. I had to lay face down and put my head in a hole that looked something like where you would lay your head when you are getting a full-body massage. She also told me that I would not be able to move a muscle for the next forty-five to sixty minutes. *Are you kidding me!* The whole process was starting to get a little too hard!

I started crying like a baby and telling the lady that I didn't want to do the procedure. I didn't want to have Cancer, and I definitely didn't feel like trying to fight it! I wanted the whole thing to be over with. *God, why me?*

That poor lady didn't know what to do with me. She asked me if I wanted her to call my doctor to prescribe me something to help me to relax, and if we should reschedule the MRI for another day. "No," I told her. "The faster I do the MRI, the faster I can be scheduled for surgery to get this tumor out of me!"

Most people would probably say that the reason why I lost it is because I had an anxiety attack. No, that was not why I lost it. I lost it because that was the first time that the diagnosis became real to me. It was the first time that I had gotten angry and cried about it.

I finally calmed down and laid down on the skinny table inside the MRI machine. The machine was extremely loud even with the headphones that they gave me. The headphones played music in an effort to drown out the noise of the machine, but they were not much help at all. I started worshiping and talking to God, and that is what got me through the procedure. When the test was over, the lady had to wake me up because the peace of God had allowed me to rest.

The next few weeks were full of doctor appointments with my breast surgeon and a plastic surgeon. I received the results of the Comprehensive BRAC Analysis test. I was happy and relieved to tell my daughter that the type of Breast Cancer that I had was not hereditary, and that she did not have to be scared about developing Cancer later on in life. In between doctor's appointments and tests, I tried to live my life as normal as possible. My supervisors at work were awesome to me. They were very flexible with my schedule and very understanding. They honored my wishes of not sharing my diagnosis with the rest of my team. I chose not to share my diagnosis with my team because I didn't want anyone to ask me how I was feeling every five minutes. I didn't want people to feel sorry for me or treat me differently. I wanted to laugh and joke with people at work like I always did. I needed my life to be as normal as possible. I worked out every day like I did before the diagnosis. I may not have been able to stop Cancer from growing in my body, but I damn sure could control how I chose to handle it. I was not going to let Cancer control me or my life.

It seemed as if it took my doctors forever to agree on a surgery date to perform a double mastectomy on me. I chose to do a double mastectomy because the last conversation I had with my surgeon resulted in her telling me that she would not be able to remove all of the Cancer with just a lumpectomy. The results from the MRI showed some smaller tumors in my right breast that I was not able to see or feel. She also stated that the lump that I was able to feel was too close to the skin. However, there was no Cancer in the rest of my body. So, when the doctor stated she needed to do a mastectomy on my right breast, I told her to go ahead and take them both.

There was no sense in having one perky breast and one saggy one. *LOL!!!* Now, there were some positives of having a double mastectomy. Once my breasts were reconstructed with implants, I would never experience saggy breast ever again. My breast would always be perky! *Oh yeah!* I also would never have to purchase or wear another bra again. Well, at least that gave me something to look forward to.

My breast surgeon's nurse finally called with a date for the surgery. My surgery was scheduled to take place on September 11, 2012. *I know...right?* What are the odds that my surgery would be performed on the same day that such a tragic event took place in America's history. Well, the idea of having surgery on such a memorable day made me just a little nervous. Oh well, I was just happy to finally get a date for surgery. Even though the doctor told me that the type of Cancer that I had was slow growing and non-aggressive, I still wanted it out of me ASAP! I was so happy that I had Lonnie as a friend, and the ladies at the workout class. I spoke with Lonnie and Kim on almost a daily basis. I would call or text them often; sometimes late at night when I needed someone to talk to because I was scared or didn't understand something that the doctor tried to explain to me. Kim was still battling her Cancer, but she was still able to keep me encouraged.

One day after workout class, Lonnie and Kim were telling me about what food to eat and not eat to help protect my healthy non-Cancerous cells. They told me to eat lots of berries; especially blueberries and blackberries because they were high in antioxidants. The funniest thing happened to me when I got home. My husband met me at the door with a smoothie made out of blueberries, blackberries, strawberries and bananas. I was like, *Wow! How did he know?* I love him so much!

Cancer Was OUR Blessing

God was a major part of me getting through this difficult time in my life. My Pastor would pray for me. I would go home and stand in front of the mirror and repeat the prayer back to myself. I was speaking to my spirit and my body. I would curse the Cancer at the root. I would command it not to grow. I would tell myself that I was healed from the crown of my head to the bottom of my feet. I also had a favorite scripture that I would read often and speak it over myself. Psalms 103:1-4 always reminded that there were benefits in the Lord. The scripture reminded me that it is God who healeth all diseases. I love God, He is so awesome and truly worthy of all of my praise in the good and bad times.

The Susan Komen Breast Cancer 5k run and walk was taking place only a few days after my diagnoses. I normally run it, but decided to walk it that year. I saw the daughter of a close friend of mine. She had been diagnosed with Breast Cancer while she was pregnant, and she was there with her baby and husband participating in the walk. I gave her a hug, and told her how awesome she looked. I then told her about my diagnosis. She gave me another hug, and told me that I would go through the necessary treatment and would be fine. I totally believed her because she looked good. I saw several people that I knew. I even saw my friend Rhonda that I had met at Lonnie's. I spoke to her and gave her a hug. As she turned and began to run, I looked up and noticed my name on the back of her shirt, along with a few other names. She was running for me. *How could you not want to fight when you have people like Rhonda who was a three-year Breast Cancer survivor at the time, wanting you to win?* My husband's family decided to form a team that year in honor of his aunt Debbie who had died of Breast Cancer years ago. At the end of the race, the Ogletree family formed a circle around me and began to pray for me. I was a little embarrassed because I was the center of attention, but I was very grateful for the prayers and the fact that they cared enough for me to do it.

Cancer Was OUR Blessing

The night before the surgery, my husband and I stopped by Lonnie's house. She wished me well on my surgery, and kissed both of my boobies goodbye. *LOL!* My surgery was scheduled for 9:00 a.m., and I had to be at the hospital at 7:00 a.m. I had already done all of my blood work the week before. I had one more procedure left before the mastectomy was to take place. I still had to have some type of radioactive dye injected under my right arm so the surgeon could see my lymph nodes. They always check your lymph nodes to make sure there is no Cancer in them.

It is the difficult times that show you how much people really care about you. My daughter told me upfront that she was not going to school on the day of my surgery. My brother Howard (Buggie), my mom and dad, my mother-in-law, my Pastor and his wife (Sister Morton), members from the church, Lonnie, Amanda, Tonya and her husband, and my wonderful husband Awri all were with me. My friend Tina, and Adrienne and her husband, came later on that evening. They were all there to wish me well, and to keep my family encouraged. I am so thankful for them.

The surgery was scheduled to be six hours long. My Pastor prayed for me again before I went in for the surgery, and I knew that everything was going to be okay. The surgery consisted of my breast surgeon going in and removing all of my breast tissue. Once the breast tissue was removed, my plastic surgeon came in and placed the expanders in along with some drains; one on each breast that would remain inside me for the next two weeks. When I woke up from the surgery, I remember feeling an excruciating pain in my chest. I heard the nurse ask me if I wanted some morphine. I heard my husband tell me to tell them yes, so I nodded my head yes. I then looked at my husband and asked him if they had found Cancer in my lymph nodes. He gave me a kiss and told me that no Cancer was found in my lymph nodes. The doctor had removed two lymph nodes to be sure. My friend, Gail, called to check on me, and to see if it would be okay for her to visit. The morphine hadn't kicked in yet and I was still in a lot of pain so I told her no.

After everyone left, the nurse came in to show me and my mom how to take care of the drains. She told me that I would have to empty them three times a day, and keep a record of how much fluid was collected. The biggest challenge after surgery was trying to get out of the bed to go to the bathroom. I couldn't use my hands to push myself up to get out of the bed without feeling a lot of pain, so I had to use my core to sit myself up. Just another reason to make yourselves do all of those sit ups that Lonnie makes us do in class, ladies. *LOL!* Once the pain was under control, my mom and I actually had fun enjoying each other's company.

I was released from the hospital the next day to start the road to recovery. I chose to spend the majority of my recovery time at my mom and dad's home. My husband would visit me every day. Lonnie, Nika, and Isha helped out a lot with my daughter, Triniti. They made sure that she worked out every day. That was important to me because my daughter struggles with insulin resistance, which makes it harder for her to lose and maintain a healthy weight. My husband was also making sure that he attended my son's football games and kept up with his senior fees and events. I spent the first two weeks sleeping sitting up in a comfortable chair. I was not able to sleep in a bed because of the drains. After the first three days in recovery, I was anxious to get out of the house and at least go for a short walk. I did not want to allow myself to get weak, and the walks helped to sleep later on at night. I was also used to working out every day, so the quicker I could get back to working out, the more normal I would feel.

My mom and dad went with me to my first oncology appointment. I had only met with a radiologist before my surgery because at first we thought we were going to go with the lumpectomy and radiation option. My surgeon had her nurse set me up with an oncologist to talk about my treatment plan for the next five years. The morning of my appointment, I had a pity party for myself and was in a bad mood. I met with the oncologist who was a male, and of Middle Eastern descent. He was abrupt, and very insensitive. He started off by immediately telling me what he thought my treatment should be. He told me that we would do chemo and that should knock out all of the Cancer. I was totally flabbergasted! Chemo was never discussed as a treatment option. My options were, lumpectomy with radiation, or mastectomy with no chemo or radiation. When I asked him why he wanted to do chemo, he stated again that chemo would get rid of all of the Cancer. I explained to him that I had only been diagnosed with Stage 1 Cancer, and it was not considered to be aggressive. I began to cry. I had already lost my breasts, and that man was trying to take my hair too! My mother explained to him that I was having a difficult morning and was very emotional. He was so insensitive that his solution to my difficult morning was to prescribe me some behavioral health drugs. I told him again, just in case he had not heard my mom correctly, "She said I was having a difficult morning! She didn't say I was crazy!"

I left the appointment and immediately called my surgeon's nurse and told her that I wanted a second opinion because that oncologist was not going to work for me. She said okay, and immediately scheduled an appointment for me with a female oncologist for the following week.

The day got better when I went to my appointment with my plastic surgeon. A full two weeks had finally passed, and it was the day I would find out if my doctor would remove the drains from my breast. I was so excited! It meant that I could start working out again, and I wouldn't have to try and figure out every day what I could wear that would cover the drains. I was on my way back to normal. I had my plastic surgeon write down all of the things that I could do so that Lonnie would let me come back to class. I was able to do everything except for weights and pushups. I went to class that same day. Of course everybody kept asking me what the hell I was doing there, but they didn't understand that working out made me feel strong, in control, and normal.

I went back to my parents' house in a much better mood than I had left in that morning. I spent a week there recovering before I went back home. While I was there, Lonnie, Isha, Nika and Kita practically took care of my daughter, Triniti.

During my recovery time, Lonnie and Amanda would meet me and my mom for brunch. They would make us laugh so hard. My friends Tina, Adrienne and Rochelle stopped by to check on me and hang out. My cousins, Dee Dee and Lee, came to visit me as well. Those visits really meant a lot to me. The fact that my friends and family took time out of their busy schedules to come and see about me...*Priceless!!!*

The last two weeks of my recovery I spent at home. I was a little angry when I got there though, because...oh my God!!! My house was not clean. It was a hot mess! Who wants to come home to a dirty house? Really! Oh well, I took a deep breath and went to my room; even that was not worth getting upset over.

I met with the female oncologist whose clear explanation of what she thought my treatment should be for the next five years made me breathe a lot easier. She said that we would wait for the tests results to come back on my breast tissue before we would decide if chemo would be beneficial to my recovery. She did say that I would definitely have to do radiation because of how close the tumor was to the skin. Radiation would ensure that they would be able to kill all of the Cancerous cells. She would put me on Tamoxifen, which is a mild form of chemo in a pill form. I would have to take Tamoxifen every day for the next five years. Tamoxifen would not cause me to lose my hair. I was upset about having to have radiation though. The breast surgeon told me that because of the type of Cancer I had, if I did the mastectomy, I wouldn't have to do chemo or radiation. I called Lonnie to fuss about it. She proceeded to talk some sense into me. Having gone through both chemo and radiation herself, she told me that she would do radiation all day long to avoid chemo and its side effects. She helped me change my mind about the whole process. By the time I got off the phone with Lonnie, I was feeling pretty blessed that all I had to do was radiation.

The tests results of my breast tissue came back. They revealed that I would have less than a nine percent chance of the Cancer ever reoccurring in my body again. That meant that I would not have to have chemo. I was so happy, and so thankful to God that I didn't have to go through that process. However, my oncologist reminded me that I would have to go through the radiation. That same day, she introduced me to the doctor that would be over my radiation treatment.

Once it was determined that I would not have to do chemotherapy, I contacted my supervisor and advised her that I was ready to come back to work. I was pretty confident that I could work and do radiation at the same time. Before I started radiation, I went to my plastic surgeon to get my last saline injections. My plastic surgeon told me that I would not be able to get my breast implants until six months after the radiation was over, so I was going to have to leave my expanders in for over a year. That would ensure that the radiated skin had time to totally heal. The expanders were not comfortable at all, and I would have to go for six more months without being able to lie on my stomach comfortably. I know this sounds crazy, but I was worried about the saline fluid in the radiated breasts possibly boiling from the heat of the radiation.

Once they prep you for radiation, the actual process is a breeze. I started radiation on November 1st, and completed it on

December 21, 2013. The radiology department gave me a certificate of completion to keep. I was very happy to be done. I had to keep the radiated skin moisturized in order to keep it from cracking, and was blessed that it didn't crack; especially since I struggle with eczema.

Life was slowly getting back to normal. In the words of Mr. Bush (Lonnie's dad), "Life is good." I was down to two doctor's appointments every three months. I probably did push myself a little too hard by trying to do everything that I did before the surgery too soon. For example, I was training for my annual KC Corporate Challenge 5K, and woke up the next day with bruises all down the right side of my body, along with a huge lump popping out of my right side. That caused me to make a call to my doctor to make sure that everything was okay. The doctor did an ultrasound, and it was determined that the lump was an inflamed lymph node.

I had that issue pop up one more time within the same year, except I did not notice the lump. I had an appointment with my oncologist, and she felt the lump under my left arm pit. I told her that it was probably an inflamed lymph node. She said that she wanted to know what was causing the lymph node to be inflamed. She told me that she was going to schedule a biopsy and left the room to start the process. Fear quickly came over me and I began to cry. *But God!* The Holy Spirit brought back to my remembrance that I am healed from the crown of my head to the bottom of my feet. God is the one that healeth all of my diseases. God also reminded me that He did not give me the spirit of fear, but of a sound mind and body. After, I spoke all of these things out loud, I began to calm down and think positively. I did the biopsy the next day like my oncologist requested. When the tests came back, they showed that there was no Cancer in my lymph nodes. I thanked God and went on about my life.

Cancer Was OUR Blessing

Six months was finally up. It was June, and time for me to complete my final breast reconstruction. In other words, I was finally going to get rid of those hard, untouchable saline expanders. Yes! I will finally be able to lay on my stomach without my chest hurting. I went for my appointment with my plastic surgeon. He showed me the type of breast implants that he would be using. My plastic surgeon was going to be using a brand new type of silicone implant that was supposed to look more like a woman's natural breast. I was totally excited. My breast were going to be on the cutting edge of technology. I was going to be one of the first people to use them. The new breast implants were called Natrelle 410; they were highly-shaped cohesive anatomically-shaped silicone-filled breast implants. The breast implants even have their own individual serial number. *Wow!* The doctors and nurses lovingly refer to the new implants as Gummy Bear implants because of the shape and the consistency that they have.

July 31, 2013 is when the final reconstruction was complete. It was a much happier occasion than the double mastectomy. I wasn't even nervous. I was just happy about getting the softer implants in. My immediate family was there for the big event. When I woke up, the doctor explained that he had a difficult time inserting the implant into the right breast because of all of the scar tissue from the radiation. I told him I could tell because it totally felt like someone had been beating me on my chest. My doctor gave me my post-operative instructions, and sent me on my way. I was not able to do pushups or weights for at least six weeks. Even though I had waited six months for the skin to heal, it was still extra sensitive and could rip, tear, or crack because it was very tight. The skin did finally heal, and by October, I was finally able to start lifting weights and do pushups. Once my doctor was satisfied with how the radiated skin had healed, he allowed me to schedule an appointment to get my nipples tattooed on at his office. So, that next week, I met with the tattoo artist who had perfected the art of tattooing nipples onto a woman's breast. The first time he had ever tattooed a nipple onto a woman's breast was for his mother who was also a Breast Cancer survivor. I had never had a tattoo before, and I will never get another one because it hurt. It felt like lots of needle pricks or bees stinging me. But, oh my God! It was so worth the pain. The nipples looked very real. They were done in a 3D fashion. So, if you took your shirt off and someone was walking by and just slightly glanced at you, they would not know the difference.

My name is Dana Ogletree, and I am now forty-four years old. I am a one year and seven month old Breast Cancer survivor. If it would have been left up to me, I would have never chosen to go through Breast Cancer. But it wasn't left up to me, and I had to fight that battle. I learned a lot about myself and others while fighting. I learned from Lonnie the importance of sharing my story. I didn't go through Breast Cancer for me. I went through it for others who will be diagnosed with Breast Cancer after me, so that I can identify with them, and take them by the hand and tell them not to quit that they will make it through. From experience, I will be able to help them understand how to take the treatment and everything will be fine. When a woman has been diagnosed with Breast Cancer and is trying to decide if she wants to do a double mastectomy or a lumpectomy, I will be the first to lift my shirt up so she can get an idea of what one looks like. When a woman comes into the gym after being diagnosed with Breast Cancer, I, too, will hold her hand and pray with her. It is my prayer that I inspired those women who were watching me fight my battle. *Did I do something that they can imitate or use that will help them fight harder?* I pray that I have.

Lonnie's Reflections

In Dana's story she explains how people are in your life for a reason, a season, or lifetime. I honestly believe God put her in my path to encourage and force her to get a checkup! Dana was in denial. She knew something wasn't right. She had blood around her nipples and she took ninety days to go back to her doctor, and just kept trying to explain it away! Friends, most of the time our bodies give us warning signs and we ignore them. We just explain them away: I'm too young, I eat right, and it doesn't run in my family! We can't let fear keep us from dealing with reality! I can't express it enough, if you don't feel that comfortable with your doctor's diagnosis, get another opinion. No one knows your body like you do!

Sometimes even the strongest warriors lose the battle. We may never understand why their time here with us was so brief; all we can do is thank God that we were able to cross their path.

Alexis Louise Wright

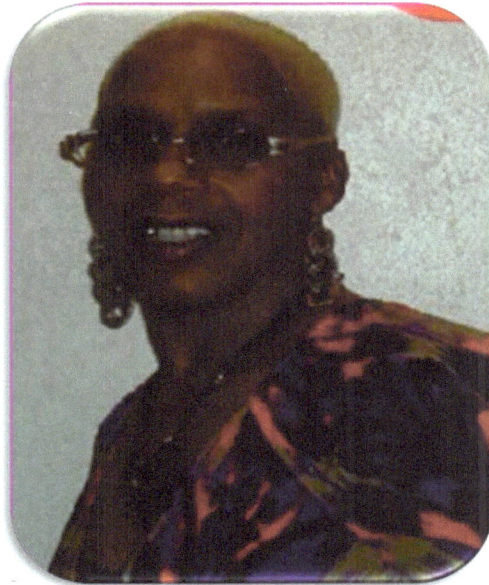

Alexis Louise Wright lost her battle to Gallbladder Cancer at the age of fifty-eight. She was a very loving mother and grandmother; a very straight forward person who always spoke her mind, and would give anyone the last of what she had. She was very giving and was as down to earth as they come. If she was your friend, she a true friend; if she wasn't your friend, she didn't pretend to be. She never was fake or phony. I remember being at work and a woman came up and was starting a conversation with Alexis. Before the woman could say more than a couple of words, Alexis said, "Girl, why are you over here talking to me? You know I don't fool with you."

I laughed so hard and asked Alexis why she said that. She replied, "Yolanda, I'm just real; if I don't fool with a person it's as simple as that!"

I can honestly say that's what I loved about Alexis most is that she didn't pretend. She was exactly who she was. No masks. No pretenses. Just Alexis. She had a huge heart, she would do things as small as bring magazines so we would have something to read when the line was down, or something so thoughtful as to bring the whole line cookies. It's times like those that I think of and start laughing. When she was ill, she wouldn't allow me to see her. In my heart, I know it was her way of wanting me to remember her the way she was, not the way she appeared. She will forever be my crazy, sweet, friend, and I miss her!

Kim Stone-Wells

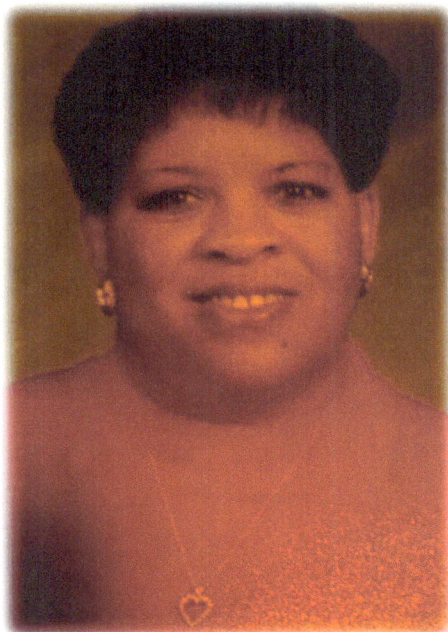

Her Faith Was Her Legacy

Kimberly Stone (Wells) was born in Sylacauga, Alabama on September 24, 1961. A Southern Belle who took care of herself, and quite often took care of everyone else, Kim always treated people right; even when they took her kindness for weakness. As is the case with most Southern girls, she could cook; and cook she did. Kim and her sister spent many hours on the phone comparing recipes and talking about new dishes. Kim is the mother of three beautiful children; Michael, Anthony, and Brandy. She took pride in her children, and raised them as conventional Southern children; very respectable and well mannered. Yes, ma'am, and no, ma'am were instilled in their core, and they have raised their own children the same way. In 1991-1992, Kim moved to Kansas City, Missouri with assistance from her sister and brother-in-law who drove her there to begin a new life. I'm not sure if it was known then, but the move was laying the foundation for many lifelong friendships.

Kim was the epitome of a hard worker. When she first arrived in Kansas City, she sought employment. Her first job was at a nursing home. Kim decided she was not cut out for the job, and would search for other means of employment on her off days. It was no surprise that she received a response to an application she submitted, and was hired and began working at Hypermart USA: a grocery and general merchandise store under one roof located in south Kansas City. She worked years of long hours and different shifts. She was determined to purchase her own home, so along with working at Hypermart, she started working a part-time job at Burlington Coat Factory. In her quest to have one job after realizing two jobs were for two people, and with the help of a good friend at her local church, Kim became employed by Peterson Manufacturing where she met and was blessed with new lasting friendships. She loved her job, and took pride in her work. She drove a forklift, and she operated it like nobody's business.

Kim wrestled with several health issues, but the most intense was her esophagus. She had difficulty swallowing. Kim knew eventually she would need to have surgery. After the matter did not improve, it was recommended to her that she have an esophageal dilation; a procedure to widen a narrow part of her esophagus. Over time, it became difficult to lock in a surgeon locally. It was suggested that she travel to Chicago, but Kim was a good steward of her money, and she didn't see the point of traveling there. After doing some extensive research, she was able to find a local surgeon to perform the procedure.

Kim often thought her other health issues – back problems and acid reflux – were connected to the trouble with her esophagus. Before she was admitted to the hospital to have the esophageal dilation surgery performed, she thanked God it was not Cancer that was destroying her body. Kim was prepped for surgery, and all anyone could do was wait. Her surgery was performed on April 5, 2013. The surgery bypassed the anticipated time and I received a call from Ericka—Kim's niece, that Kim was out of surgery. There was a long pause. I waited for her niece to tell me that Kim was in recovery, but to my dismay, I was told the surgeon found Cancer. Having surgery is one thing, but to come out of surgery and to hear that the anticipated surgery was not performed because when she was opened Cancer was present, of course, that was unsettling; it would be unsettling for anyone. Calls were made to those close to Kim. She had a very supportive church, and her church family was very helpful; not to be outdone by her coworkers. Kim's children all lived in Alabama and were told the news by telephone through their Aunt Shelia.

Kim was not told right away. The initial procedure wasn't done, and Kim had been heavily sedated. It was decided to tell her the news once she was stable and the anesthesia had worn off. Once Kim was alert, the news was given to her. She was taken aback. Her first thought was of how her dad had died of Cancer. When she was told, she responded, "I'm going to suffer like my dad." Following the doctor's news and discharge, Kim wasn't big on talking about her diagnosis. She was in disbelief that she had Cancer. *Baffled!*

After meeting with the oncologist, a treatment plan was scheduled. The oncologist decided to attack the Cancer aggressively. The treatments seem to do well until the last treatment that was scheduled ended up being cancelled. Kim was too tired and weak; the oncologist decided against another treatment at that time. It was recommended that she retire from working and file for disability. Kim was completely against it. She was determined to go back to work. Her body grew tired, and she ended up yielding in to retirement. She was determined to overcome the setback of Cancer, to be healed, and to return to work eventually. Kim had worked all of her life, and it destroyed her to not to be working.

Cancer Was OUR Blessing

Kim was admired by her children for her work ethic. No matter how sick or how much pain she was in, she went to work and worked her butt off, even when she was told she wouldn't work anymore because of her recently diagnosed Cancer. Kim was determined to show the world that she would return to work. Brandy, Kim's only daughter, considered her mom to be simply amazing, and often said she wished she could be as strong mentally and physically as her mother was.

As time passed, Kim experienced a great deal of pain in her stomach. It was so painful that she found herself bent over while going through it. Kim looked at the pain as being the Cancer leaving her body. She was a woman of faith, and remained in prayer. She knew God was sovereign, and nothing altered her faith. She stayed positive. She was determined to fight, and under no circumstances was she going to give up.

Kim did everything within her power to move forward. When talking to family, she asked what else could be done. Eventually, the doctors on staff said there was nothing else they could do, but Kim said, "That's their word, not God's Word, and I don't believe them." She could not believe this was the expected end and she was not alone. We were all in shock. Kim continued to stand firm and trusted in the salvation of God. When she was discharged from what she was told at the hospital, getting Kim to talk was not easy. We practically had to force her to talk.

Her eating habits changed considerably. She said nothing tasted the same. Her taste buds were intensified; salty things were more salty, and the sweet things were even sweeter than she remembered.

Thanksgiving rolled around, and to her surprise, Kim was blessed with an airline ticket (roundtrip) from her co-workers to visit her sister in North Carolina. Although she was extremely happy to visit her sister and brother-in-law, Kim wasn't feeling her best prior to boarding the plane. After the plane ride, she began to feel even sicker. Upon her arrival to her sister's home, there was soup prepared by her brother-in-law. She ate a little of the soup and said it was good. During her entire visit in North Carolina, Kim was moving slowly; not to mention the fact that she ate very little. Her sister knew something was wrong, but Kim exclaimed she was fine. That's how Kim was. She preferred not to be fussed over. She always thought of others first and herself last. Kim didn't want to disappoint her sister and disrupt the Thanksgiving dinner that was planned.

Time came for Kim to return home. When returning to Kansas City, she had a connecting flight and while waiting for a wheelchair, Kim became sick; very sick while in the airport terminal. The vomit was dark black, possibly the sign of old blood. After she feebly stood in the women's restroom cleaning herself up, she boarded the plane and finally made it back to Kansas City.

Cancer Was OUR Blessing

When Kim's niece and her niece's husband picked her up, Kim began to vomit uncontrollably along the highway; the same black vomit. Even though Kim requested to be taken home, Kim's niece, Ericka, knew Kim needed to be in the hospital. Without hesitation, they drove Kimberly to the hospital emergency room.

Kim insisted on the doctors doing everything in their will to help in the healing process, but there was nothing they could do. The doctors had done all they could, and told Kim the same.

Kim looked at the doctors and asked, "Am I really dying?" Her faith was her legacy. She believed in God for a complete healing. She never gave up. She fought to the very end.

Brandy will never forget that; never for a second did her mom give up in believing that her God would heal her until she was wrapped safely in his arms.

I received a text from Brandy at 5:49 a.m. on December 31, 2013 saying, *Mom is unresponsive again. Nurse on the way.*

At 6:11 a.m. I told Brandy I was on my way.

January 1, 2014 at 4:48 a.m. Kim passed away. She had twenty-one grandchildren.

~ Shared by Shelly; friend

Lonnie's Reflections

At times, stories like Kim Stone's confuse me. I say, "Lord, she fought so hard to stay alive to beat Cancer, she didn't just give up!" Then I have to remind myself that we don't know what the person was praying. Also, we all have to eventually leave this earth. We belong to God, and He calls us home when our time is up. It should not matter how we die more that it matters how we lived.

Prior to the end, I went to see Kim and she was up and talking. She smiled and said, "Hey Lonnie, you finally showed up," we both laughed, and a week later she was smiling with the Lord!

Aliyah Rachelle Spann

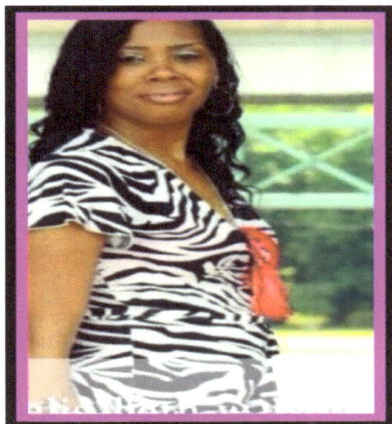

Aliyah was only forty-two when she lost her battle to Cervical Cancer. Knowledge is key with Cervical Cancer as it can be treated if caught early. As she fought her battle, Aliyah wanted women to know how important screening is for early detection, and the reality that clinics provide tests for those that are uninsured. Aliyah stayed positive and had a smile and laugh all the way to the end.

~ Shared by Fatima Spann, sister

The Faces of Cancer

There are more than one hundred different types of Cancer. Those afflicted vary in age, sex and race. Although there are some risk factors which can attribute to some forms of the disease, Cancer does not discriminate. It does not see color or economic status. It could care less about one's position in life.

The faces of cancer come in all shapes and sizes. Education, prevention, and treatment are its enemies. Faith, encouragement, and support are its friends.

Cancer Was OUR Blessing

Jan Blackstock

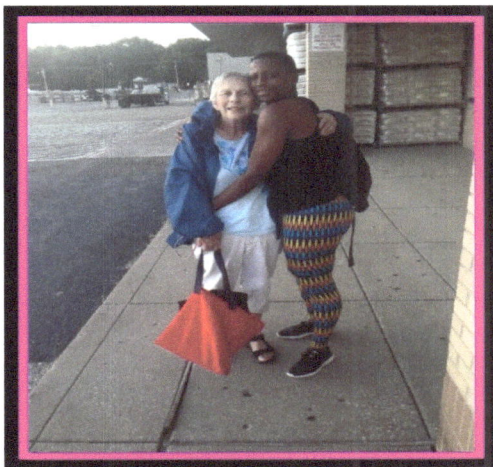

I met this beautiful lady at Walmart, she worked in the plant department. Never in a million years would I have imagined she would become my friend and leave such an impact on my life! Through conversation between two strangers, we discovered that we both battled Triple Negative Breast Cancer; the most aggressive form of Breast Cancer that there is. Mrs. Jan and I went for rides and had long conversations. She never complained, not even when her Cancer returned as Stage 4 in her lungs and bones. She decided to enjoy her life to the fullest for as long as she could, and not to go through treatment for a second time. She traveled and went to places she had always wanted to go. She tried restaurants she had always wanted to eat in, and experienced things she had never experienced before. The return of her Cancer sparked something inside of her that encouraged her to enjoy life with every breath that she took until she could breathe no more. During our last moments together, she looked at me with tears in her eyes and said, "Lonnie, I'll miss you, but I'm kinda excited about this journey!"

Mrs. Jan left Kansas City and went to pass peacefully surrounded by her kids and grandkids.

Cancer Was OUR Blessing

Claudia Sandoval-Radillo

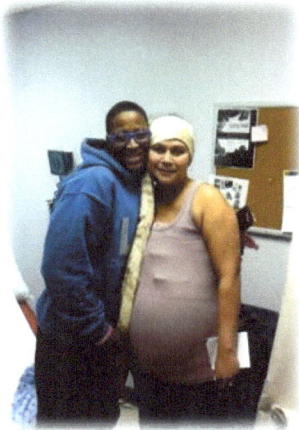

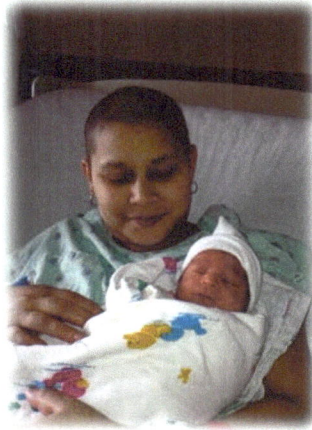

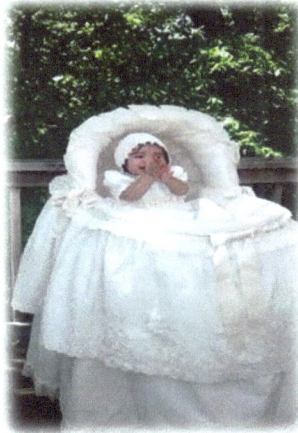

I met this beautiful lady at the Cancer Center. I noticed she was pregnant, wearing a head scarf, and her breast was missing! I was heartbroken. She was busy fighting for her life so that she could enjoy the life she was carrying. Claudia was very soft spoken as she informed me that she already had five other children, and was on birth control at the time that she became pregnant. She said that she and her husband had decided not to have any more children after the birth of their two year old. Their children range in ages from two through twelve years old. Claudia also informed me that she was shocked to learn of her pregnancy because she was on two different forms of birth control. She was even more shocked to learn that she had Breast Cancer and needed to start treatment immediately.

The pregnancy, although unplanned, was a miracle because it saved her life. It was the reason all the prenatal exams were done and the Cancer was found. After initially meeting Claudia, I noticed that I hadn't seen her at the Cancer Center in a while. I later found out that she was missing appointments because she didn't have the finances to pay her copays, or to afford the gas to get back and forth for treatment. Can you imagine not being able to show up for the treatments that you need to save your life, simply because you can't afford gas or copays? I asked the patient navigation supervisor, Tina, to check all of Claudia's upcoming appointments which required a copay. Tina gave me a printed copy of the upcoming appointments. I, in return, gave Claudia the funds for all remaining appointments that required copay and I gave her a gas card. I made her promise to keep all of her appointments.

Claudia also shared with me that she didn't have a car seat to bring the baby home in. I reached out to friends and did a fundraiser. When it was over, I met Claudia again and delivered a car seat, stroller, clothes, diapers, and everything that the baby might need. She looked at me and started crying.

"I don't understand why you're doing this!" she said as the tears ran down from her eyes. "It's what the Lord left me here to do!" I replied.

I'm proud to say that Claudia gave birth to a beautiful, healthy baby girl, and she is done with treatment and is Cancer free! One person can make a difference; that person can be you!

Janice Wells

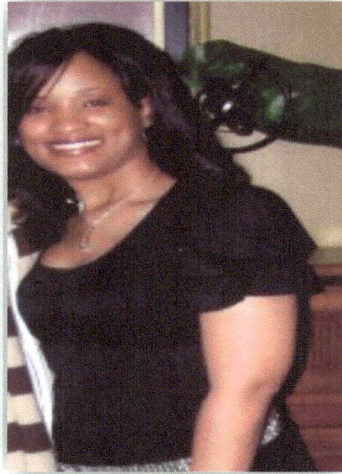

Beautiful on the inside and out, Janice never let anything dull her radiant smile. She was thirty-five and left us too soon when she lost her battle to Medullary Carcinoma of the thyroid. Janice graduated from Baker University with a BS in Business Administration. She was a mother of three who loved them with every bit of her being until she took her very last breath. She was a great friend to all who knew her, and she always greeted you with a smile; even while she was dying.

~Shared by Nori Wells, husband

Nikki Carmouche

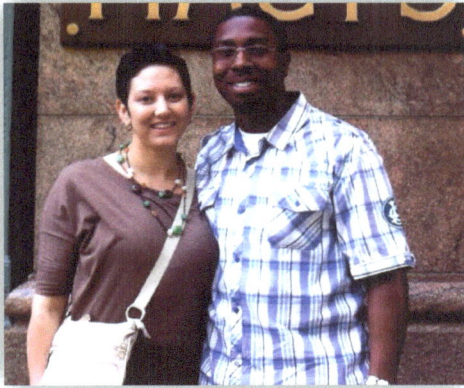

Nikki's Journey

My name is Terrell Carmouche and this is the story of my late wife, Nikki Carmouche. I still cannot believe she is no longer here with me. My days are tough, but my children give me the strength I need to carry on.

Tanikka (Nikki) Joy Gambirazio Carmouche, was born April 17, 1981 in Cherry Point, North Carolina, to Ms. Debra Licari and Mr. Fernando Gambirazio. Nikki was a graduate of Havelock High School, Class of 1999; she went on to obtain an Associate's Degree from Craven Community College. While living in Havelock in 2005, Nikki met a Marine who would two years later become her husband, Terrell Carmouche. In her spare time, Nikki enjoyed scrapbooking, selling Scentsy, and interior decorating.

In 2009, two months after the birth of Nikki and Terrell's twins, Nikki noticed a grape size lump on her right breast. Nikki decided to go to her doctor to get the lump checked out. After conducting a basic breast examine, the doctor decided the lump was a swollen milk duct due to the recent birth of the twins. Nikki went home with instructions to pump more milk, massage the area, and apply a warm rag nightly. A few months went by, and the lump increased to the size of a golf ball. Back to the doctor again she went, and again, swollen milk ducts was the diagnoses. Nikki continued the heavy massaging, increased milk pumping, and application of a warm rag.

In May of 2010, finally after the lump grew to almost the size of a grapefruit and displayed signs common to Breast Cancer, Nikki went to seek a second opinion with a Cancer specialist. She was tested, and when the results came back, Nikki was diagnosed with Stage 4 Breast Cancer. She was devastated due to the fact that she knew when the lump was grape size, that something was seriously wrong. She was even more devastated at the fact she put all her trust in one doctor, and he was wrong. After a double mastectomy, a lumpectomy, radiation, and months of chemo, Nikki appeared to be Cancer free.

In late 2011, Nikki noticed pain coming her right pelvic area and lower back. After some tests were done, it was revealed that her Cancer had returned; but this time, it had spread to her pelvic, lower spine, and some other organs. Nikki was informed she needed to start radiation immediately on her spine, and she underwent a new round of chemo.

By mid-2012, the doctor noticed the current chemo medication wasn't working like before. He decided to switch her to a different one, but after a while, the results were the same. The Cancer had begun to adapt to the new chemo. Nikki tried every chemo she could, but the Cancer was so aggressive that the results only lasted for six weeks at a time. As the Cancer grew in 2012, Nikki was given one year to live.

In 2013, Nikki started having severe pain in her side and difficulty breathing. It was determined that the tumors in her lung were weeping, causing fluid to buildup in the lung. That required Nikki's lung to be drained. Months later, the lung would fill back up; each time with more fluid. The doctor decided to install a drain into her side to help her drain the lung. During the summer of 2013, due to an increase in fluid in both lungs, Nikki was told she only had two months to live. She decided to seek a third opinion.

In August 2013, Nikki was accepted into the Cancer Treatment Centers of America in Philadelphia, Pennsylvania. The treatments they decided on for her, were the same as her local doctor. Nikki decided to only travel to CTCA for her testing and her six-week treatment. Her second round of treatment at the CTCA was a tough one due to the fluid in her lungs. Nikki decided that traveling to Philly was too much on her weak body, and since the prescribed treatment was the same, she would just stick with her local doctor.

Early in October 2013, with friends and family accompanying her, Nikki met with her doctor. He informed us all that she was down to only one chemo option, and that was only to buy a little more time. The doctor asked, "Do you want to try this and feel sick, or would you rather enjoy what time you have left?" We all agreed it was best to enjoy the time.

Early in 2014, the Cancer started making normal life more difficult for Nikki, so she started hospice care. On February 16th in the blink of an eye, Nikki took a turn for the worst. She had difficulties communicating and became bedridden. Within two weeks, Nikki was unable to stay awake for more than a few minutes a day, and was unable to leave the bed. Her pain was growing, and so were her struggles with breathing. Her pauses between breaths became longer, and with each breath you could hear the fluid inside her lungs.

Nikki lost her courageous battle with Breast Cancer at her home on March 5, 2014. She was surrounded by her loving family. She touched countless people from all walks of life with her infectious personality. Nikki's funeral was the biggest that her church had seen in over fifty years. Cars lined up on both sides of the street and up and down every alleyway. Her hospice worker came to the funeral and told the story of when she first met my wife.

Nikki had told her, "You know you're going to cry for me."

The case worker said, "I've been around for a while and I've seen a lot, but I will be sad."

After talking about the person she met, and had grown to love, and telling the story of what my wife had told her, the case worker cried.

Nikki always had a smile on her face and never let what she was going through show on her face. She was an angel who walked amongst us; a wife, a mother, a daughter, a sister, a friend, and someone who there will never be another like again.

~Terrell Carmouche

Lonnie's Reflections

Like a lot of us, Nikki trusted her doctor. Most doctors treat all patients the same. I've met countless women for whom Cancer could have been diagnosed sooner if the doctor would have done testing instead of writing it off as swollen milk ducts. Nikki went from a grape size lump, to a golf ball, to a grapefruit. We must always seek a second, third, or even a fourth opinion if needed. At times, we have a feeling that something is wrong, but we want to trust and believe our doctors.

Nikki fought a hard, brave, courageous fight that could very well have been won! When you finish this story, say a prayer for her husband and family.

Cancer Was OUR Blessing

Shawna Caruth

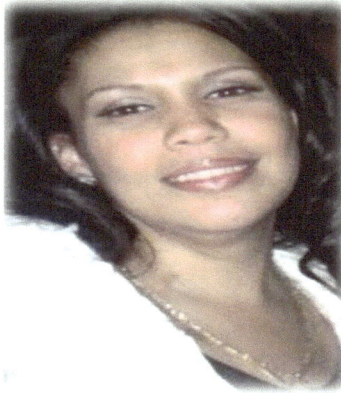

Dignity, grace, and class can only begin to describe Shawna. When diagnosed with Uterine Cancer, doctors gave her six and a half months to live, but God saw fit to bless her with seven and a half years. Before her passing at the age of thirty-five, Shawna touched many lives in many different ways. A true supporter of family and friends and very strong willed, she always kept her head held high, accompanied by a bright smile.

What I will remember most about Shawna was that she always said, "Thank God for every day; good and bad."

~Shared by Cia Houston, cousin

Cancer Was OUR Blessing

MiMi French

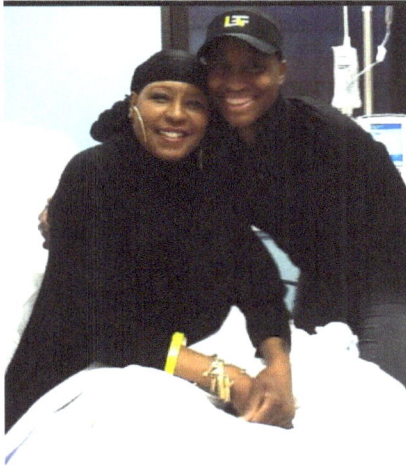

New Beginnings

I felt the lump, and then I acted like the lump was nothing for about seven months. At a doctor's appointment, I asked my doctor to feel the lump. I was told that it was nothing to be concerned about, and that it might just be a fibroid or something like that with a much fancier name. I even asked a few family members and friends to feel the lump as time went on as well. I was concerned, but everyone seemed to think it was nothing to worry about. When I was in the hospital for my Congestive Heart Failure, a tech had the OB on staff to look at the lump and that doctor said it really did not feel like nothing to concern myself with, but he said if it was bothering me that much, that I should get it checked out.

Well after all the time that passed – I'd say maybe a year, and the fact that I had let so many friends and family look at the lump, I named it Herman. I kept hearing about Breast Cancer and finding out that a few of my friends had recently learned that they have the big C and were starting their own battles. I was so nervous, but I went to my doctor and she set me up for a mammogram…

Ok, and so it began. I was so nervous, yet convinced that God would give me a clean bill of health, so I held my head up and my mother and I went in for the exam. After the exam was done, I instantly asked the tech what he thought. Now keep in mind, a tech is NOT A DOCTOR…

He said, "Well, do you want me to give it to you straight up?"

I said, "HELL YEAH, that's why I asked."

I just knew he was going to give me good news because he is only a TECH, not a DOCTOR, so he couldn't possibly see anything bad.

He went on to say, "Ma'am, if you don't have God in your life, then I would suggest that you do ASAP."

I replied, "Yes, sir, I have a personal relationship with Him, THANK YOU VERY MUCH!"

He said, "Well, I've been doing this for over twelve years…" he may have actually said more years than that, but I kind of blocked that part out, "…and I am a Cancer survivor and I know that this is exactly what I am looking at on this report."

My mind was in disbelief and I thought to myself, *Well, sir, I am happy for you and I will pray for you, but what in the HELL does that have to do with me? I'm different.* I told the tech, "Thank you very much," and we left.

Cancer Was OUR Blessing

It was the longest week to follow, waiting for the report to come back. *Well, GOOD MORNING to me.* I looked at what had arrived in the mail. It was a letter about the mammogram, and on the report it said in so many words that I needed to see my doctor ASAP because I had a lump. *Well, DUH!*

So I started praying and telling myself that this would not happen to me because it's not what God has in store for me; plus He spoils me, and oh yeah...I'm different. Okay, so moving along, I went to the Women's Breast Clinic *BY MYSELF* because I was so sure that everything was going to be just fine; after all...I'm a nice person, I love everyone, they call me Mother Love, I have a personal relationship with God, I am a single mother, I'm trying to get my life together for me and my son, I'm a great person, and I have way too much going on in my life to deal with BC. Hell, I have heart problems to deal with already, not to mention nobody in my family has, or had, Breast Cancer. From all of that alone, I knew I had nothing to worry about.

The doctor came in the room with me, and we remembered one another, so we spoke on a first name basis. As we laughed and went down memory lane (I told you everybody loves me), we finally got down to what I came in for.

He says, "Undress and put this gown on, we are going to do a biopsy. It really does not look like anything to be concerned about because it's moving some, and Cancer doesn't move."

I got undressed and went to the other room where they did the procedure. I should have taken someone with me, is all I could think about. After the biopsy was performed, I went back to the first room with my head held high because I already knew my report was going to be different.

Cancer Was OUR Blessing

When the doctor entered the room, as soon as he sat down and crossed his legs, he said, "Ms. French, the report is back." When he called me by that name I knew then that something was wrong. We had left on first name bases, and he came back with *Ms. French*. Hmmm.

I replied, "Okay, since we're being professional now, yes doctor, what's the news?"

"You have Cancerous cells," he stated as a matter of fact as he kept on talking. I could not hear anything else that came out of his mouth until he said, "Do you have any questions?"

A tear fell down my eye and all I could say was, "Call my mother or my sister."

I don't remember much else except the fact that somehow I managed to fill out paperwork and make a follow up appointment. But other than that, I really can't tell you what was said to me after that. I just kept telling myself that I would be okay because I was different. Then I did the humanly thing to do...I cried.

I'm not going to take you through the whole story step by step but just know I cried, was sad, got angry, mad as hell, oh yeah...and did not understand why this happened to me. Oh, and I kept questioning the universe as to whether or not I was going to lose all of the hair that was down my back that I love dearly because it made me so much prettier. My mind was spinning out of control. I had a son, was a single mother, I'm not a bad person, no one has had Breast Cancer in my family, I cry when I can't help others, I pray for single mothers at the bus stop, I give anyone my last...I am different! *WHY ME?*

Meanwhile, back to the story...I was diagnosed with Invasive Ductal Carcinoma Breast Cancer. They did not tell me the million dollar answer of "WHAT STAGE" until I had the surgery. Herman (the lump) was very close to my heart, so the doctors had me do chemo first to shrink it before they would even try to remove it. That was a safety precaution. Chemo was the worst thing I have ever had to deal with in my entire life. I thank God for my support team. Without them, I would not have made it. I was also given radiation to help keep the Cancer away. So after all of this, it was time for the big surgery. Let me be the first to tell you that I was not only excited about getting it over with, I WAS SCARED. They performed the surgery and you will never guess what the report was...they had removed the scar tissue from where the lump (Herman) was located and six lymph nodes. The tissue came back NON-CANCEROUS and all six lymph nodes came back Cancer free! I was told that this was an amazing report, and that I went from Stage 3 to a negative 1. It's as if I never even had Breast Cancer.

I AM DIFFERENT.

As I rock my bald head, I'm learning to love myself even more. The journey is not over yet. I'm currently doing chemo and radiation, but when it's all said and done, I kicked Breast Cancer in the ass.

Lonnie's Reflections

Just like in MiMi's case, many women ignore symptoms as if they will go away simply because they choose to ignore them. Well, that's not the case, that's sets us up for higher Stages, harder fights, and sadly...deaths. Sure, in a perfect world we would all like to hear the words, "You don't have Cancer." Sadly, we all don't. So wouldn't you rather hear, "Yes, you have Cancer, but we caught it early and beating it is attainable," than hearing, "It's a late Stage" or "It has spread, and the chances of beating it are slim."

MiMi beat Cancer. Her hair is growing back, and she still rocks!

Kimberly Jones

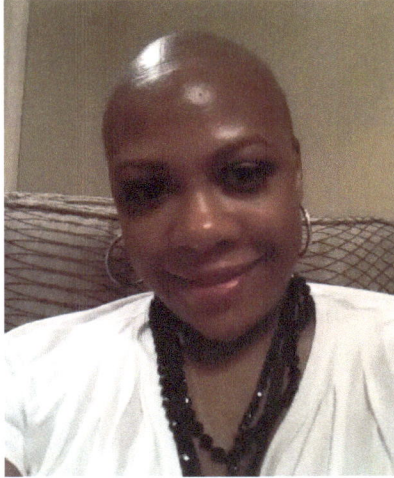

Pink Chose Me

In my eyes, my life was going pretty good. I was thirty-five, had married the love of my life, had a baby, my daughter was becoming a young lady, and I moved into a beautiful home. I mean what could go wrong; right? October 2012 I received the phone call at 7:00 p.m. that every women dreads.

"You have Breast Cancer."

I couldn't respond the way I wanted to because I happened to be at my sixteen-year-old daughter's school event, and she was sitting right next to me when I received the call. I didn't want to alarm her of the news I had just received because as a mother, you want to protect your children by any means necessary. Imagine having to sit through an entire program after receiving some news of that magnitude. I was completely numb.

Cancer Was OUR Blessing

After the program, I rushed home to give my newly-married husband the news. I told my daughter to go upstairs to her room, and I closed the bedroom door. I sat next to him, tears running down my face, and told him the doctor called me with my test results from my biopsy.

He grabbed my hand and said, "Tell me what she said." I didn't have all the details yet, so I told him exactly what she said. "

They found a *small* amount of Breast Cancer in my right breast." My husband threw my hand away, flared his arms in the air, and fell out on the couch "Aww nah!" he repeated. I looked up at him and began to laugh so hard. This time I grabbed his hand and assured him that everything was going to be ok. For the next year, everything I went through, he went through.

After I had my son in 2011, I went in for my routine checkup. I told my doctor that while breastfeeding, I felt a knot in my right breast and it had been bothering me and would become sore at times. She gave me a breast exam and assured me it was a clogged milk duct. I was told to come back in six weeks if it did not go away. Six weeks came and went, and so did my health insurance, so I did not go back to the doctor. I wasn't too concerned about the knot because the doctor seemed pretty confident that it was only a clogged milk duct from breast feeding. A year later, it was time for my yearly exam and I had medical insurance once again. I made an appointment to see the doctor, and while having my exam, I brought it to her attention that the knot I had shown her last year was still there. I will never forget the look of horror that was on her face as she examined my breast. This time, the confidence she portrayed the year before was replaced with fear and concern. As she was making my appointment for a mammogram, she tried to stay calm and tell me that she still didn't think it was anything, but I knew different.

My life would be changed forever. The next day, I went in for my mammogram; at age thirty-five, it would be my first. It was a little uncomfortable; especially on the right breast where the knot was. They said I had some suspicious areas that they wanted to biopsy. A couple of days later, I went in for the procedure. I was put in a room with a monitor, and given the choice to watch them suction the area, but I chose not to look. At the end of the procedure it was confirmed. I had Breast Cancer.

I was sent to a Breast Cancer specialist where I found out what type of Breast Cancer I had. I was told I had Stage 0 Ductal Carcinoma. The specialist told me I would only need to have a lumpectomy. I mentally prepared myself for a lumpectomy. Before I had my procedure, I had to go in for a MRI. I was put in a long tube and had to stay really still. My husband was in the room with me, and placed his hand on my leg for the entire ordeal. He knew how afraid of closed spaces I am, and just knowing he was there helped me to relax.

The nurse came in after they were done and told me that she would send my results over to the specialist. I knew something was wrong when she came in that room. I could feel it. As I left she said to me, "Good luck."

I look at my husband and said, "Good luck? What does that mean...good luck? Why would she say good luck?"

I just rambled on in my head trying to analyze the look on her face, and the action of her placing her hand on my shoulder as she left the room. Something just did not feel right.

I went on to see more specialists and have more testing done. I had a genetic test done; you are rated from 1-34, 34 being the highest of the Cancer to return and 0 being less likely. My test came back at 20. That meant I would have to have chemotherapy; at least it would be in my best interest. Next was radiation. I would have to go for radiation every day. Everything was just going so fast. I would write down questions for each doctor because by that time I had seen four different doctors.

I was still going to work every day; it helped me keep my mind off of everything that was going on. One day as I arrived at my job, I received another phone call from the doctor's office. After reviewing the MRI, they noticed that the Cancer was a lot deeper than what they originally thought. My Stage 0 was now Stage 1, and I would have to have a mastectomy. I cried hysterically because I had only prepared myself mentally for a lumpectomy, radiation, and chemotherapy. Now they were telling me I would have to have my breast removed.

I opted to have a bilateral mastectomy to lessen my chances of the Breast Cancer coming back. I also would not have to have radiation. November 9, 2012 was surgery day. Mentally, I was at peace. I can honestly say I never asked God why. I only asked God to give me the strength to help me and my family make it through. It was like having a baby; God gives you a nurturing spirit when He gives you a baby. When I had to go through the storm, He gave me a peaceful spirit. I knew I was going to be ok.

All of my family arrived at the hospital and they had the lobby packed. They came into the room one by one to show their love and support. I had not cried all morning until my uncle walked in the room. I hadn't seen him in a while, and all of a sudden, I was overwhelmed with emotions. Everybody that showed up had such a special place in my heart, and I couldn't thank them enough for being there.

The anesthesiologist came in and I was ready for my cocktail. I remember being rolled down the hall to the surgery room with my family behind me; they walked as far as they could with me, but this was a journey I had to take all by myself. Waking up in the recovery room, I felt like I had been hit by a diesel. I had never experienced that type of pain before. I was released from the hospital the next day. The pain was so intense that I could not stand or sit up straight. I slept in a lazy boy chair for at least three weeks. They sent me home with tubes coming out of each breast to catch the remainder of the blood. I would have to have the tubes in until all the drainage was gone. I cringed when I had to empty my drainage tubes because I hated the way it smelled. It was a stale smell; a smell of sickness.

I remember being bandaged, and afraid of looking down at what use to be my breasts. I finally mustard up the courage to peek, and what I saw were these odd shaped, no nipple, breasts that were as hard as a brick. I can say that I was a little disturbed by the image of the new me, but after I took my pain medicine, I forgot all about it. I had tissue expanders placed in to stretch out my skin to get ready for reconstructive surgery, but that would not happen until after chemotherapy months later. I felt like I was going through an outer body experience. It just didn't feel like I was in my own body. I would still have a smile on my face; mostly because it didn't feel real.

I made it through surgery, which was a physical challenge; but the real challenge would start after chemotherapy, because that was more mental. I started chemotherapy a few weeks after surgery. I really didn't know what to expect. Yes, they talk to you before you start, but you've talked to so many doctors by that time, that everything starts meshing together. Every third Wednesday, I had infusion, which is just another term for chemotherapy. That went on for the next four months. In between going to chemotherapy, I saw my reconstructive surgeon every Monday to have saline put into my tissue expanders. I hated going because they would take a long needle filled with saline, and insert it right into the center of my breast. Having reconstruction surgery after a mastectomy is different from reconstruction for any other reason. The difference being that you are cut straight across the breast; they cut your nerves. So I no longer had feeling on the top layer, but I could still feel the needle on the inside.

The first day of chemotherapy was a long, tiring day. I was there for about four hours because they had to run test before they gave me my treatment. After my first treatment, I felt fine. I thought they all would be a piece of cake. The next day, I was still feeling good; but by the third day, I started feeling the effects of the treatment. My body started aching; eating was difficult because nothing sounded good to eat. The chemotherapy had taken away my taste buds.

A week or two went by, and I was taking a shower when I noticed my pubic hair coming out. By the time I got out of the shower, it was like I just had a fresh wax; I mean completely bald. That wasn't so bad until I noticed the hair on my head started coming out as well. My friend and co-worker, who also was diagnosed with Breast Cancer two weeks after I was, had our hair braided before surgery. I remember sitting on the couch and braids would literally fall out of my head. One day I went to the bathroom and cut all the braids out. Cutting the braids as low as I could, my hair was still coming out in gobs. I would pull on an area and be in shock of all my hair coming out. I started having bald spots all over my head. I called my cousin who is a barber, and asked him to shape up what little hair I had left. It looked nice, but it was not low enough. My hair continued to fall out, so I told my husband to get the clippers and to skin me bald. After he did, I could not look at myself in the mirror. I immediately told him to put a hat on my head as I tried to fight back the tears. For the entire day, my daughter and husband tried to convince me that I looked fine, but I did not feel fine, and I slept in my hat until the next day when I had enough courage to look at myself.

The image of me was no longer me. By that time, I was completely bald, my eyebrows and eyelashes were gone, and I had picked up weight from the steroids. I remember walking by a mirror and having to do a double take because I did not recognize myself. *Who was the person starring back at me*? On the inside, I still felt like me; but the outside told a totally different story. I was watching TV one evening, and one of those commercials came on that showed people being in the hospital sick from Cancer and I began to weep because I said, "Lord, that is me." It was one of the hardest things to do...to see yourself change right before your eyes and not be able to do anything about it.

Another side effect from the chemotherapy was that it put me in a medically-induced menopause. It was twenty degrees outside, and I would be in the bed with the fan on, the window open, and butt naked. That was definitely, in my opinion, one of the worse side effects I had to deal with. I remember being at the mall with my wig on, and a sales lady was talking to me. I could feel a hot flash about to start and sweat started rolling down my forehead from underneath the wig. I snatched that wig off in the middle of the store, took off my coat and scarf, and told her to just give me a minute. The lady stood there with her mouth open in disbelief, but I did not care because when those hot flashes came, they came hard and I would dare anybody to say anything.

It's hard to believe it has been a year since my chemotherapy. The road to recovery has not been an easy one, but I've had so much support to help me through it. I thank God for my family and my family in-laws who have made sure everything around me was taken care of; all I had to do was focus on getting healthy.

Yes, PINK chose me, but I did not let my circumstances dictate how I would live my life.   If I had one thing to tell women, it would be to know your body. Get checked; early detection is key.

Lonnie's Reflection

At the end of Kim's story she said *early detection is vital*; sometimes early detection makes the difference in your treatment plan, and certainly in your chances of survival. Ladies, handle the diagnosis differently; the first step is accepting the reality that you have Cancer, which can take a while to really set in. Then comes the task of how you tell loved ones and giving them time to accept it. Another thing positive about Kim's story is that she had support from family and friends. A lot of women don't have that, and have it helped Kim keep a positive attitude.

There are times in life when we have to go through ups and downs; and some of those ups and downs are inevitable. You might as well go through it with a positive attitude, because being negative won't change the situation, but it can change the outcome. Your body is going to fight stress or fight to get well!

Cancer Was OUR Blessing

Karen McNair

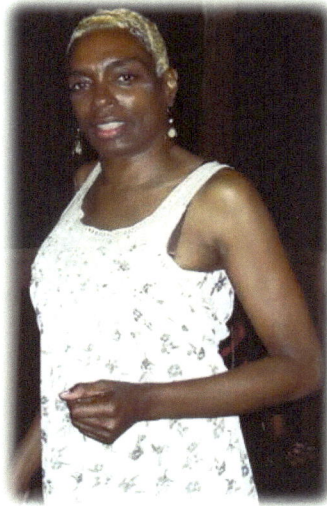

Unshakable Faith

My name is Arthur Jackson Jr., my friends and family call me Jap. Karen McNair was my fiancé' and this is her story.

When I first met Karen, we did not have time to date. I honestly believe that God placed me in her life to walk with her on her journey.

From the first day I met Karen, I stayed with her every day until the Lord called her home.

How is this? You ask. Keep reading, because I have a story to tell.

I walked into my sister Rosalind's beauty salon one day, and she asked me was I still dating my ex-girlfriend. I let her know that we were no longer dating, and that I was a single man. I was actually looking for a mate. She told me she had the perfect person for me to meet. She asked me to take this girl's phone number and call her. I refused. I told her I was not calling any strangers and then I added, "BUT! You can give her my number, and she can call me."

Carla, Karen's best friend, showed up just as I was walking out of the Salon. Rosalind ran out the salon to meet Carla to tell her that I should meet Karen. They described Karen to me, and told me that she was a great catch. I told them to simply give her my number.

Well, they gave Karen my number. Two or three days after Valentine's Day 2009, Karen called me. We had a great conversation over the phone and then I asked her when I could meet her.

She said, "What are you doing now?"

I said, "Nothing right now."

She said, "Come over later on this evening."

I went over there, and she remembered me from when we had danced together at a nightclub years prior. While sitting in the kitchen talking, we really hit it off.

I went back the next day, the day after that, and the day after that...so after a week, I moved in with Karen because we got along so well. There was no sex, and I was cool with that because I was celibate myself. This is why I feel that our relationship was the work of God and He knew what was about to happen to Karen.

Karen lacked affection as a child, and I gave her that. I know she loved me. I sometimes feel that she loved me more than I loved her. She treated me like a King and she was my Queen; we were good together, she loved her some me. We had great times talking and getting to know each other. She would always make my favorite dish of spaghetti and salad, and she would cook it just like my mom cooked it. Karen also loved God very much and lived her life according to His Word. She prayed in her lavender and purple prayer room. She had a prayer team called, *The Prayer Warriors* and they would be in prayer every morning at 5:00 a.m. praying on the phone.

She never pressured me about going to church; but eventually I started going to church, praying, and reading the Bible with her.

I took Karen home to meet my parents, and my sister Rosalind was over there visiting. When I attempted to introduced them they already knew each other from school. When I introduced Karen to my mother, she called my mom Momma Barb. My mom loved it, and they shared an immediate bond and talked like they had known each other for over twenty years. My mom knew there was something about Karen that was special. *Why?* Because over a short two week period of time, I moved in with her. LOL...but if my dad tells the story, he would say that it was an overnight move in.

One afternoon, we were listening to the radio and they mentioned something about *Take your bra off Thursday*. I started teasing Karen about her bra, and that's when she told me that she was a Breast Cancer survivor. Then she asked did that bother me and I told her no, not at all. She said it bothered her ex-husband which caused them to divorce. He could not handle her sickness. I reassured her that I had no problem with it.

One day in May 2009, Karen came to me and said that her side had been hurting. She took some pain medication and it stopped. Two weeks later it came back and we were expecting out-of-town guests. The pain was still there, yet she managed to entertain them. Karen went to the doctor and they ran some tests, but she felt that they ran the wrong test, because they determined the pain to be arthritis and they started her on steroids to ease her discomfort.

We took a trip to Phoenix and Karen was miserable the entire four days. We made a doctor's appointment immediately when we returned to Kansas City. Karen found out that she had Bone Cancer and it was in her hip and that had metastasized to her lung. The surgeon suggested that she get a hip replacement to remove the Cancer from the hip before they started any type of chemotherapy or radiation treatments for the rest of the Cancer. The surgery was performed in November 2009.

Karen had to learn how to walk all over again with the assistance of her friend. One day, she took the walker away from Karen while at the mall, and she made Karen walk without it. She began walking very well and never looked back.

Later, Karen was strong enough to start the chemo and radiation treatments. In the beginning of 2010, we made many trips back and forth to the doctor and to the Cancer Treatment Center. That is where we met Lonnie Bush. I had known Lonnie from years ago from our old neighborhood, but Karen and Lonnie clicked instantly because they were really loud talkers. They began to chat, and Lonnie gave Karen hope, along with many ideas about how to maintain her health throughout her treatments. They would also meet up to walk at the local park. Lonnie would come in the Cancer Center with gifts for the patients. She would pass out hats and scarves to those that were battling Cancer. The center would even announce that Lonnie was there to help. This made Karen love her new friend, Lonnie Bush, even more. Lonnie gave Karen a few scarves and stocking caps.

As I stated before, Karen and I really didn't get a chance to date because the Cancer came in and it was aggressive, so she went through a lot of sickness which caused some ups and downs for us. I got frustrated with the Cancer, not with Karen. All I wanted to do was just help her. I wanted to take the Cancer away. Karen asked me to leave her three times, but I couldn't do it, so we cried together and I promised her that I would never leave her.

As the time went by, Karen got stronger and was able to return to her job while she was getting treatments because she was placed on a chemo pill. She worked for the IRS and things got better with her health. It was time for my annual Phoenix trip, and Karen went with me again, yet she was in pain, but not as much pain as the year before. She continued to battle, and then they found three spots on her brain in November 2010.

Karen never complained and she always put her trust in the Lord. There was a time where she did get weary and refused treatments, and they called me in to assist her. In my heart I believe they gave Karen some news about her condition and she didn't want me to know. Karen tried to prepare me that she was not going to make it in a subliminal way; but I trusted God for her healing.

In January 2011, Karen wanted the living room painted and asked her close friend John to come over and paint. He and his wife (also named Karen) came over on the 29th of January 2011. Karen was weak that day and was not able to make it downstairs to see his work, but she had a great conversation with John's wife.

She was developing a cold and I brought her cold medications that she needed. Later on that evening, I sat on the side of the bed and began to cry because I wanted to take the sickness away. I felt as if I wasn't doing enough for her.

She replied to me and said, "You have done yours! Everything is going to be alright!"

Cancer Was OUR Blessing

I felt much better and went downstairs. When I came back to the room, Karen had changed clothes; she had on a black blouse and black Capri pants. She was wearing all black.

She was sitting in the chair and I begged to take her to the hospital. She told me that she was not going back to the hospital because she didn't need to. She went on to say that if she needed to go back to the hospital that she would let me know. We talked, then I went downstairs again. She got back in the bed and went to sleep. She looked so beautiful. I went and got a cool towel to wipe her face and she loved it. I tried to give her the medication and she refused it. She asked me to put on her favorite CD, but to turn the volume down low. I did, and went back to my man cave downstairs. I told her that I would be back in an hour. When I came back upstairs, Karen appeared to be sleeping well.

I sat down on the side of the bed and said, "Baby, take this medicine," and her arm was cold. I lost it. I called 911 and they assisted me over the phone with performing CPR. The paramedics came, but they could not revive her.

My fiancé was gone, but she left this earth in peace.

In my heart, I think Karen wanted me to leave the room so she could pass on.

God got His glory by getting me back in church, reading my Bible, and my praying. I send prayers out to all my friends and family ever since Karen has been gone. I started sending inspirational messages and scriptures a few days after her funeral service, and I have not stopped.

I thank God for choosing me, I really do. I have no regrets. I just wish she could have beat it, but in my heart I know it was God's will.   I love you Karen.   Your King, Jap

Lonnie's Reflections

Arthur said God placed him in Karen's life for her journey. I'm a firm believer that God places people in our lives for a reason, a season or a lifetime! Karen was so motivated to get better; never once complaining or doubting God. Her faith was unshakeable regardless of what she was going through. I walked into the chemo room one day, and heard someone talking and laughing loudly. I thought, *Who is that? No one disrupts the treatment room but me!* I found out it was Karen; she was battling for the second time. Her first battle was with Breast Cancer; the second battle was Bone Cancer that would later spread to her brain. My spirit and Karen's spirit connected as soon as we met. We talked like we had known each other for years. We exchanged numbers because as my fight was ending, hers was starting again, and I wouldn't be on the chemo injection side anymore. I would be on the side that administers radiation. We talked on the phone and through text messages.

Karen was trying to gain her muscle and strength back, and also trying to put her weight back on. We agreed to meet at a track close to where we both lived. While we walked and did squats, after every lap, I noticed her getting short of breath and asked her if she wanted to take a break. She informed me that her lungs were damaged from all the treatments and it caused her to get short of breath quickly. I must have expressed a look of sympathy because she said, "No, you not gonna look at me like you feel sorry for me. I see the way you push your clients, don't treat me any different!" she continued, "I trust God no matter what happens in my life. I don't trust doctors, I trust God!"

We walked around a couple more times with Karen wheezing the whole way.

After that, Karen was getting stronger and wanted to go shopping for jeans, she said, "I wanna get my weight back so I can look good for my honey!" I was finished with treatment and back to my busy schedule. Karen called because we setup a date for me to go help her pick out jeans. I missed the call. I later returned her call and got her voicemail. I laid down to take a nap. Karen called twenty minutes later. I figured I would call her after I woke up and set up another date to go shopping. Sadly, two weeks had passed, and I hadn't called her back to reschedule our date. I had an appointment the following week at the Cancer Center, and figured Karen and I would talk, laugh, get caught up on things and if she felt up to it go find her some jeans.

I received a call from one of my favorite nurses from the Cancer Center, she said, "Yolanda, Karen's husband asked for your number, but because of patient confidentiality, we couldn't give it to him, so we took down his number to give to you."

I took his number, wondering what it was that he wanted, but I didn't get around to calling to find out.

It was Friday morning, I tried to make all my appointments for Fridays. I walk into the Cancer Center, and I could feel the nurses looking at me, but I brushed it off to them just not seeing me in a while. I walk in the back to where I always donate hats and scarfs. I kinda laughed because almost all the scarves that I left my last visit were almost gone.

I looked at one of the nurses and said, "Karen must have been here because the scarves are gone." Karen loved my scarves, she would even take the ones I wore on my head.

The nurse looked in my eyes and said, "Yolanda, you didn't call Karen's husband did you?"

"No," I replied. "I figured I'd see her today."

She walked close and touched my arm and said, "Oh honey, we tried to get a hold of you, Karen passed!"

Her lips were moving, but I was in a state of shock, like time was standing still. When I opened my mouth, the tears began to flow. I said, "When are her services?"

The nurse looked away from me and replied, "The service was almost two weeks ago."

I couldn't hold back any longer, I stood Karen up. I didn't return her call. I didn't call her husband. I didn't know she passed, and I didn't get to even make peace by attending her service! I couldn't get out of the Cancer Center fast enough! I was devastated. I sat in my truck wishing I was dreaming, wishing I could wake up and take her shopping, wake up and visit her at home when she got sick, wake up and at least attend her funeral services. But it wasn't a dream, and I felt horrible. I had put something off that I could have made time to do, and now I would never have the opportunity to do it. I'd pushed someone away because of my own circumstances. I sat in my truck in front of the Cancer Center and I cried, I prayed, I reevaluated my life! I realized that everything we go through isn't for us, but at times for others around us.

I agree with Arthur that Karen had made her peace with the Lord and waited until he left the room before she walked into the arms of the Lord! I struggle daily with not being there for Karen. It's the reason I started *Celebration of Life*. I want to make a Cancer patient's fight easier. I want to encourage them. I want to assist them with anything they may need. This assignment the Lord has me on is tough. It's emotional. I lose sleep. I get down at times. I use my personal funds when I have no donations. I never would have chosen this assignment for myself.

Although it's impossible to assist everyone that comes my way, I strive to assist all that I possibly can. Whether it is a phone call, a text message, an inbox message, a hospital visit, or funeral assistance, my greatest fear is hearing again, "Yolanda, you are too late!"

I can't save or assist the whole world; but in my heart, I want to assist all that I possibly can.

CLOSING REMARKS

My friends, life is going to seem unfair at times, it's going to throw us some curve balls, it may even devastate or shock us, but God knows all and He knows the path our lives will take. Nothing is a surprise to Him! No matter how tough life gets, allow nothing to steal your joy. Yes, through trials, situations, setbacks, let downs and even Cancer, you can have joy. No, you cannot achieve it without a relationship with God, and joy, peace, and understanding come from God; ask Him for it.

Early detection is vital; get checkups if you're not comfortable with the results or recommendations from a doctor, and always seek a second or third opinion if needed. Cancer does not discriminate, it doesn't care where you live, work, your age, or your nationality. My life's mission will always be to encourage early detection and to do whatever I can to make someone else's fight easier.

Friends, you have to turn your *Trials* into your *Testimony;* share it with others, and don't keep it to yourself. To all the families that have lost loved ones, please remember you may have been praying for them to be healed, and they were also praying to be healed, well...God answered your prayers, and it may not have been the answer you wanted, but friend...they are healed and free of pain. They are absent from the body, but present with the Father. Amen!

Celebration of Life is my nonprofit organization. I pay copays, buy headscarves and medications for Cancer patients. I also assist with transportation to doctor appointments, school supplies, and Christmas gifts for kids whose mothers are battling. God left me here to do a job, and that is what I intend to do, and it is not limited to assisting with funeral arrangements.

Donations may be made to
celebrationoflife@lonniebushfitness.com

Cancer Was OUR Blessing

Don't wait until Cancer touches close to home before you decide to help!

To all my beautiful sisters that fought hard all the way to the end. God bless you…

Shawna Caruth
Linda Grayson
Karen McNair
Kim Stone Wells
LaTonya Colbert
Nikki Carmouche
Aliya Spann
Janice Wells
Jan Blackstock

Rest well, you have earned the greatest reward!! See you all when I get there.

www.ingramcontent.com/pod-product-compliance
Lightning Source LLC
Chambersburg PA
CBHW041217270326
41931CB00001B/7